Relax She's Natural
The Reintroduction

Relax She's Natural
The Reintroduction

Copyright © 2023 Deanna Browley
ISBN 979-8-9895355-0-7

All rights reserved. No part of this publication may be reproduced, distributed, or transmitted in any form or by any means, including photocopying, recording, or other electronic or mechanical methods, without the prior written permission of the publisher, except in the case of brief quotations embodied in critical reviews and specific other noncommercial uses permitted by copyright law.

For permission requests, write to the publisher,
addressed "Attention: Permissions Coordinator" at the email address below.

relaxshesnatural@gmail.com
Printed in the United States of America

Published By
Deanna Browley

Publishing Consultant & Book Cover Design

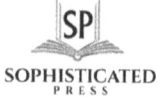

ACKNOWLEDGMENTS

Thank You, God, for giving me the vision, heart, and mind to complete this book. I am grateful for the ear to truly listen to and seek to find the truth. Thank you for planting such a precious seed, entrusting that I will bring understanding and clarity about the gift you've bestowed upon us all. I'm extremely grateful for the amazing support system you've given me, with them I have all I need to complete my assignment.

To my amazing husband, James (my strength) thank you for having faith and patience, always reassuring me that what I start, should be finished in excellence! Your unfiltered feedback allowed me to viewpoints from every perspective and find the answers myself! Your ability to think outside the box motivated me to always dig deeper. Countless nights that you kept the children occupied so that I could research and work on the manuscript. The love and support you show fuels me. Your motto that "No one is going to outwork you" replays in my mind! God, I am grateful for allowing our union.

My beautiful children Jayla, and Jaslynn James Jr. Thank you for being mommy's inspiration, knowing on many days I didn't give up, knowing that you all were watching. Your patience with Mommy while she worked on making the world a more accepting place for you. Remember to always remain confident in who you are, for every part you were fearfully and wonderfully made.

DEDICATED TO MY MOTHER:

Wylee Mae Williams

Thank you for my first encounter with the world of beauty. I remember watching you apply your makeup, spray your favorite perfume, and being amazed that all you had to do was apply water to your hair to activate the most beautiful profound curls! Long or short, your various styling choices were always of great beauty and poise. I truly never knew a love like yours before. Your wisdom, strength, and sense of humor are embedded in me. You were my very own Captain America, my shield and security blanket! Your transition from your physical form to spirit has been less than ideal, but I've chosen to continue my race. No one told me that the most important job of a superhero was to prepare their protege. Well, Mommy, I'd like to say,

Thank you for a job well done...

I LOVE YOU

Deanna Browley

Table of Contents

Introduction............................... 6
Separation 9
Reconstructed 14
Origin...................................... 19
10 STEPS 23

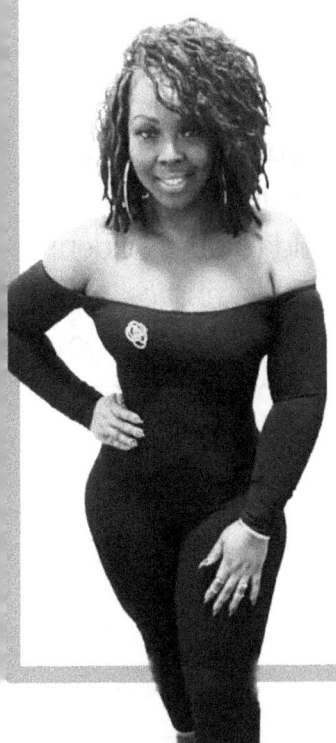

INTRODUCTION

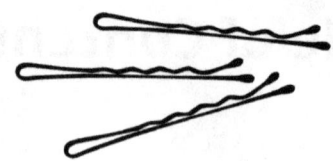

I've spent years providing services to Black Women who were confident in every major aspect of their lives. Ranging from the careers they wanted to pursue, the homes or neighborhoods they'd like to live in, down to the number of children they wanted to birth. I mean they were truly impressive and highly educated professionals who held high-ranking positions within their companies. So imagine my surprise when I started to notice one thing they all seemed to have a common.

When the decision had been made to embark on a journey of embracing their natural hair over ninety percent were underwhelmed with the reflection they saw. Quite naturally the wheels started to turn, and I asked myself what is the disconnect? Many times Black Women are told to be confident and embrace their natural hair, but how do you embrace what you don't know? How do you embrace a part of you that you haven't seen in so many years that you have no recollection of it?

The Re-introduction wants to offer a fresh perspective of psychological disposition that is often left out of the equation when Black Women decide to embrace their natural hair. What poses to be a difficult task for women in general, is magnified times ten for women of color! For hundreds of years, a Eurocentric standard of beauty was pushed, leading to generational scars so deep the effects are still felt to this very day! The more women I encountered it became evident to me that I had to help re-establish relationships! It hit me that, the majority of these women haven't seen their natural hair in decades, so indeed that reflection that stared back at them was a stranger!

Who will the book help?

The grandmother taught her daughter that you need to "Grease" your scalp for your hair to grow. The daughter went on to teach the granddaughter that thick-full hair means nappy or difficult and needs a "relaxer". To enlighten an intrigued colleague, you shouldn't attempt to pet a person's hair even if "you asked". Assisting the "eye witness" in identifying the real perpetrator. Most Importantly the woman who is searching for validation to love the reflection she sees in the mirror.

YOUR BEAUTY IS SUFFICIENT

How will the book help?

It will reconcile the relationship between black women and their hair serving as a facilitator to change and acceptance! Providing an opportunity that was taken away from them so many years ago.

Re·in·tro·duc·tion
/ˌrēəntrəˈdəkSH(ə)n/

noun

: the action of bringing something, especially a law or system, into existence or effect again.

SEPARATION

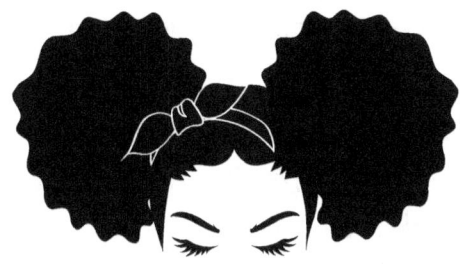

August 1995, Summertime Chi, was filled with Ponytails and Bolos, Braids, Daisy Duke shorts with white tennis shoes, Freeze-Pops, and Quarter-Waters, it also went down in history as one of Chicago's hottest summers to date! It was Wednesday afternoon, and my mother had just permitted me to go to my best friend's house to go swimming. The development she lived in had the BEST pool, it never failed to have an abundance of cute boys! I was excited to show off my new one-piece swimsuit (I wasn't allowed to wear a two-piece). FINALLY, I made it to her house we changed into our swimming clothes and headed straight to the pool! Just as I thought, people young and old had the same agenda that day, which was to cool off!

I was having a ball so it didn't hit me until it was too late, that I had immersed my entire head in the water doing a cartwheel in the pool! Oh NO, my hair was going to look like one big tight afro, but my fear was short-lived when I was suddenly distracted by my friend's smooth silky hair... but how?

I had to learn the magic secret that had been done, how was her hair straight coming out of the pool and then she uttered the four-letter word that changed my life forever. "Girl, I have a PERM," a "Perm" what's that? My mother mixes the contents that come in a kit and then puts it on my hair. I couldn't get home fast enough to ask my mother if she knew what it was and most importantly could I have one! I wasn't in the house five minutes before yelling out "Mom, can I get a PERM?" "Once you turn 13" she replied. We were only allowed to wear braids or press & curls.

My countdown began instantly. I would be free from tangled hair kiddie barrettes, infamous four ponytails, and lastly that DREADED hot comb. I even made up a little song for holiday hair:

"Twas the night before Easter, and all through the house, you could hear faint cries of little girls saying ouch."

Getting this perm became an obsession for everyone finding out who had a perm. I learned to perm quickly (or so I thought) and could always tell by how sleek the hair was after styling. Getting a perm was going to open everyone's eyes to how beautiful I TRULY was. It would cover my forehead so that my pretty smile and eyes would be the focus.

It was clear to me, people found naturally curly or naturally straight hair more appealing, and mine was neither. My hair was the least curly of my six siblings, see I didn't get the "Good Hair" gene. I've always paid attention to hair even at a very young age, I remember one time, it was my sister and I bath time, and her hair would get wet and have the prettiest curls! I would think why doesn't my hair do that because we are sisters? There are times strangers would say how adorable she and her hair were but when it came to me crickets. That was about to change because I just knew the "perm" was going to solve all of my problems! Having straight hair all the time, I'd have more confidence, more of an identity and it'd be clear just how beautiful I was.

A young black girl growing up in low-income housing had additional pressures to look and play a certain part. Everything had to be on point, clothes and shoes had to be in season, and fly hair was a must! It took what seemed to be a lifetime but finally, my thirteenth birthday was here, just in time for my party at Rainbow Roller Rink on Saturday! My mother had made it in from work and it was finally time for my life to change. The box was green with yellow and black it read, African Pride "No-Lye Relaxer" regular strength one complete application! My mother followed the directions and proceeded to apply everything to my hair.

I could feel my hair getting smooth by the second, but then it started to tingle and burn. If that's all I had to endure to have beautiful hair then it was worth it.

She rinsed the perm out completely, shampooed, and conditioned it with products from the box. It was styling time, so excited to see the big reveal only to be met with one of the greatest disappointments in my life, I was looking at one of the most pitiful ponytails and bangs I had ever seen. I remember thinking this isn't what I expected at all, my hair wasn't as long as I had anticipated but at least it was straight, right? Not at all!

My hair did not meet the requirements for NONE of the 8th grade's most popular hairstyles! The irony to this fiasco is the style that worked for me was box BRAIDS. All of that to end up back at square one. Every phase of life revealed a new insecurity that was anchored deeper than any root within my hair strand. It was never enough, whether curly, straight, long, or full, I always felt inadequate.

To think this all started from what I believed would be the answer to my prayers, it was more like the beginning of a nightmare. Years spent seeking validation from family, peers, and colleagues needing reassurance that I belong. Years spent investing in a version of me that would be deemed worthy of society's beauty standards. Conditioning that leads one to believe the mental, physical, and emotional tolls taken are worth the reward. Could this be true, the way Black Women wear their hair was considered a prerequisite?

Sealing our fate, so to speak ... you know? When it came to love, promotion, acceptance, and recognition.

It is indeed mind-boggling that in such a progressive society, a Black Woman's naturally textured hair is hard to accept. Could it be that we are partially blamed and leading by example? Ask yourself how we require other ethnicities and nationalities to embrace what we have yet to? The first encounter majority of black women had with their natural hair was TRAUMA. Whether it being, burned by a Pressing Comb or chemical Relaxer, too much tension from being braided, or the mental damage done to hearing, it's "Too Thick", "Too short", and "Too nappy"! Truly millions of women have been disconnected from the most authentic forms of theirselves. Coming to this realization ignited a desire within me to help every woman that I serviced and came in contact with. I learned that, unlike other ancestral traditions that had been passed down from generation to generation, the history and pride of our textured coils were not, instead polluted with fabrications.

1) When was the last time you wore your natural hair?

_____
_____
_____
_____

2) Was it by choice or alleged necessity?

_____
_____
_____
_____

RESUSCITATION

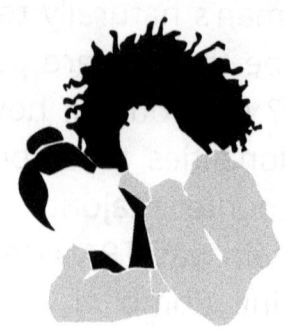

Black women are plagued daily with identity crises, the same as a child who has been abducted and separated at birth from their parents. The developmental event involves a person questioning their sense of self or place in the world. It was alarming to find that countless number of women received their first relaxers as young as 3 years old! Malcolm X once posed the question "Who taught you to hate the texture of your hair?"

I imagine it started when the Portuguese first arrived in West Africa, it was in search of gold as well as other raw materials and goods around the year 1444, and they closely observed the habits, cultures, and traditions of the African Natives. Quickly learning that hair in some cases held in a higher regard than clothing, the detailed braided styles of native people were forms of communication as well as pride. A mist early 15th century Europeans strategically shaved the hair off slaves in an effort to isolate them and strip them of any former identity, disguising it as a method of sanitation.

In reality, it was known that Ancient African hairstyles were used for many reasons, tribes often communicated Social Status, Age, Marital Status, and Religion through various intricate braiding styles.

Centuries later, here we are dealing with ideologies and beauty standards that became "New" traditions our ancestors went on to teach. Resulting in a culture of women who fail to recognize their reflection in the mirror. Convincing an entire race of their inadequacy due to their genetic traits. Years upon years of poor representation of black people have left the world to believe they're a race of filthy unattractive less intelligent beings.

The agenda was undeniably successful in perpetuating self-hate, fear, and uncertainty, causing millions of black women to believe the natural beauty they possess will always need improvement. Think back on that impressionable age where you were influenced by everything you saw and experienced. From the way you dressed, music influence, the type of food you ate, and especially how you wore your hair. In either case, how do you believe the choice impacted your natural hair journey today?

Do you suffer from any debilitating scalp disorders or hair conditions? Considering that one-third of black women are prone to develop traction alopecia, caused by excessive heat, chemicals, and tight repetitive hair styles it is safe to say yes.

In the majority of these cases, there is a lack of knowledge on both ends of the stylist as well as the client. Not to say that it is or isn't done in malice yet to shine a light on miseducation and improper technique. In this journey of recovery, it is pivotal that we begin the process of unlearning habits and traditions that no longer benefit in our overall growth. Only in recent years has a more accurate representation and proper education become a priority. If you find that hard to believe, just pay attention the next time you're at the doctor's, watching television, at the movies, or out with the family, take a glimpse at some of the most influential figures.

News Anchors, Actresses, Athletes, and Physicians are all embracing their natural tresses. Broadening the representation of endless possibilities if you choose to explore your natural hair route. For centuries the power that is associated with beauty has been withheld from the Black Woman, the architects and inspiration of the majority of the world's beauty standards. Years of cultural appropriation have diminished the peerless beauty and essence of the culture of black women to mere trends.

Alarmingly I found the majority of these women's self-value was outsourced, directly affecting the Prefrontal Cortex in the brain (where your thoughts, actions, and emotions are regulated).

Face it, women are scrutinized over the majority of their life decisions, and the thought of an unexplored version of yourself can be intimidating. Especially when knowing from where these insecurities stem. Black women make up 21% of small business owners and 7% of corporate America that being true, time management is imperative to their lifestyle demands.

We must explore the intersection of mental health and natural hair care. It should not be taken lightly, it should be approached with a patient resiliency understanding that time can heal old wounds. Start by unraveling the stigmas and create the welcoming environment that cultivates the consistent social and cultural change, you desire. Be intentional, with crowning glory. Allowing a perspective that goes beyond the mirror leading to liberation.

Welcome each strand of hair to tell its story of beauty, perseverance, and determination.

In my opinion, this mental "maintenance" practice ensures emotional balance. Shedding the weight from years of ridicule from peers in the community, professional colleagues, and some cases your own family a proper burial can promote healing.

Trying to simply forget is not enough, it will continue the cycle of women who fail to recognize their radiance and the importance of embracing it.

No one size fits all whether you decide to wear it Curly, Loc'd, Double Strand Twisted, Blown-out, Braided, Taper Cut, or Colored, no matter the direction have confidence in your destination. The strides being made in legislation with "The CROWN Act" which originated in California, is a law that prohibits discrimination based on hairstyle and hair texture, extending protection for workplaces as well as public schools, hopes the remaining states decide to follow suit. It's safe to say The Natural Hair Movement is having a moment right now!

How can this progress be seen as problematic? Well it's simple, a "moment" by definition means a very brief period, and with the history of behavior, the "moments" that took place in the early years did not sustain. It's been my privilege to experience the beauty industry as both Consumer and Professional and one thing is certain we do not want this momentum to be treated like a trend! Until the world is on board to accept hair that comes from ALL races are a genetic trait you should not be demonized for the way it grows out of your scalp.

The diminishment will not stop unless Our goal surpasses "The Natural Hair Movement. It's time to incite a Re-Introduction, one that dispels the myths and misconceptions that have been placed on a Black Woman and her hair.

ORIGIN

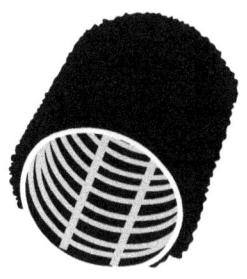

Majestically Curl'd Angel with gravity-defying Angles, tresses deemed a blessing from God the most high, as it blossoms from the scalp and grows out toward the sky. Tangible tangles sometimes accompanied by tears, are not meant to cause sorrow nor instill fear, yet to inform you that all things under the sun need water to grow, you're meant to flourish it was written, it is so.. Brown Skins girl your crown's so fly truly a chameleon it replicates fabrics ... even clouds in the sky, as whispers of judgment fill the air they don't understand the magic in your hair, The symphony of curls, cascading down with grace whirls and twirls of tresses we embrace
you are The MOVIE... STAR

A reintroduction is less about achieving someone else's #HairGoals particular look, length, or the ideal. It's focused on embracing your roots by reclaiming your natural hair. History, Strength, Sensuality Complexity, that is Beautifully Naturally known as the Black Woman!

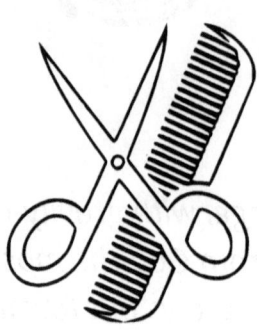

Are you ready to start your journey?

- Embrace the transition.
- Nurture your crown.
- Radiate confidence.
- Celebrate your unique beauty
- Rediscover your hair identity by debunking myths and misconceptions surrounding natural hair
- Give yourself grace and have patience through your journey of reconnection
- Embrace the versatility that your canvas allows, everyone is unique
- Nurture your mind and spirit and transition with confidence

Revolutionary in itself, intentionally breaking barriers so bold, as your curls flow with the wind your story is told.

The Reintroduction is on a mission to empower and educate black women. Creating a safe space where women of all ages and demographics feel supported and celebrated. Developing a reference point for women who desire to reclaim their identity with a fierce determination. Providing them with personalized guidance on navigating uncharted territories. While instilling confidence in women who in other words feel inadequate, resulting in the emergence of women so confident that it redefines the standards of beauty in the Black Culture.

You see for years I too pursued a relationship with my natural hair, one of rediscovery to have a deeper understanding. One that caused me to reevaluate certain beliefs I had towards myself. I realized the need was greater than a professional cosmetologist who executed a style well, but one who breeds inclusivity and the ability to cater to the diverse needs of black women. Starting with the exploration of their own beliefs, tailoring to each woman as an individual.

I'm not talking about a quick money grab by creating products and simply plastering "Natural" on the label. Nor a hairstyle that mimics natural styling that compromises the hair's true integrity.

I speak of a revolution that reunites black women with their natural hair, one that nourishes their spirits as well as their appearance! Years of these women being told that their natural hair was unprofessional, unkept, and undesirable. Taught and groomed as young girls that your God-given curls need to be tamed to fit society's narrow definition of beauty.

If ever there was a time to reconnect crown and soul it is NOW! It's time for you to take the steps of a proper introduction not one perpetuated through the narrow lens of the media. I call on Black Women around the world to allow this book to inspire you to unveil your crown with confidence and PROPER REINTRODUCE YOURSELF!

Deanna Browley

10 STEPS TO REINTRODUCING YOURSELF TO YOUR NATURAL HAIR

STEP ONE
Embracing Your Roots.

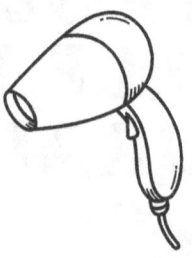

To start your natural journey, embrace the beauty of your roots. Celebrate the uniqueness of your hair texture, as it is a reflection of your heritage and identity. Let go of societal pressures and begin to appreciate the versatility and beauty of your natural hair.

DATE: _____

The last time I saw my natural hair was...

WWW.RELAXSHESNATURAL.COM

DATE: _____

STEP TWO
Educate Yourself.

Knowledge is power. Educate yourself on the various hair types within the black community and understand the right techniques and products for your specific hair needs. Research and learn about ingredients that are beneficial and harmful to your hair, so you can make informed choices. I also recommend a full blood panel this way you can truly know what's best for yooverallall health.

DATE: _____

My hair type is...

DATE: _____

STEP THREE
Establish a Hair Care Routine

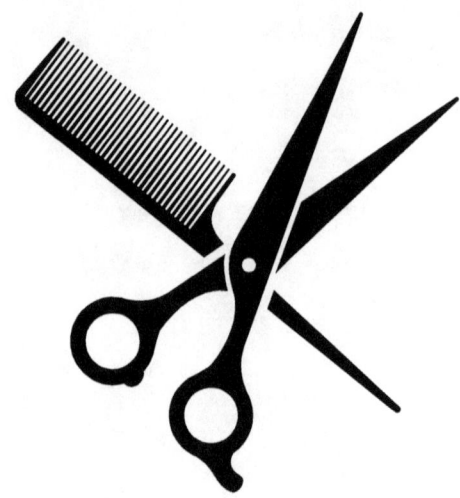

Create a hair care routine tailored to your hair's needs. Experiment with different products and methods to find what works best for you. Dedicate time to care for your hair, incorporating deep conditioning, moisturizing, and protective styling.

DATE: _____

I will dedicate the following time and day of the week to care for my natural hair...

WWW.RELAXSHESNATURAL.COM

DATE: _____

STEP FOUR
Patience is Key.

Transitioning from chemical treatments or extensions to your natural hair requires patience. Embrace the process and understand that it takes time for your natural hair to thrive. Be gentle with your mane and allow it to grow and flourish at its own pace.

DATE: _____

I understand that it is a process to transition from chemical treatments. I will give myself the proper time to transform my hair by performing the following...

WWW.RELAXSHESNATURAL.COM

DATE: _____

STEP FIVE
Find Inspiration

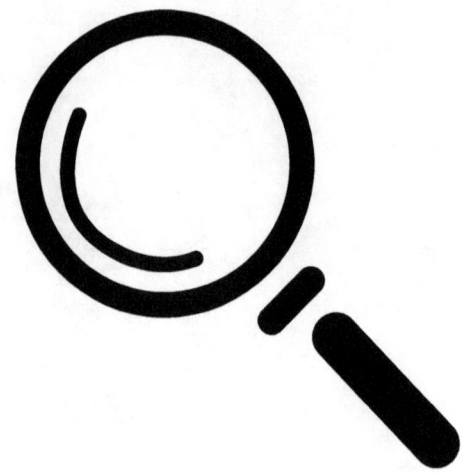

Seek inspiration from other black women who have embarked on their natural hair journey. Social media platforms, blogs, and magazines can offer valuable inspiration, styling tips, and product recommendations. Remember, everyone's hair is unique, so embrace what works for you.

DATE: _____

I am inspired by the following people who have embraced their natural hair journey...

_____
_____
_____
_____
_____
_____
_____
_____
_____
_____
_____
_____
_____
_____
_____
_____
_____
_____
_____
_____
_____

WWW.RELAXSHESNATURAL.COM

DATE: _____

STEP SIX
Nourish From Within

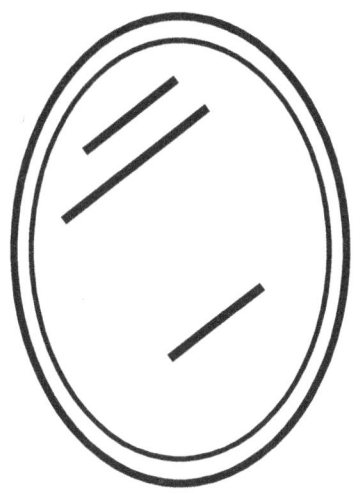

Remember that beauty starts from within. Pay attention to your overall health by eating nutritious foods and staying hydrated. A healthy diet and lifestyle contribute to the vitality and strength of your natural hair.

DATE: _____

I will commit to changing my diet so that my hair can be stronger because...

_____
_____
_____
_____
_____
_____
_____
_____
_____
_____
_____
_____
_____
_____
_____
_____
_____
_____

DATE: _____

STEP SEVEN
Experiment With Styles

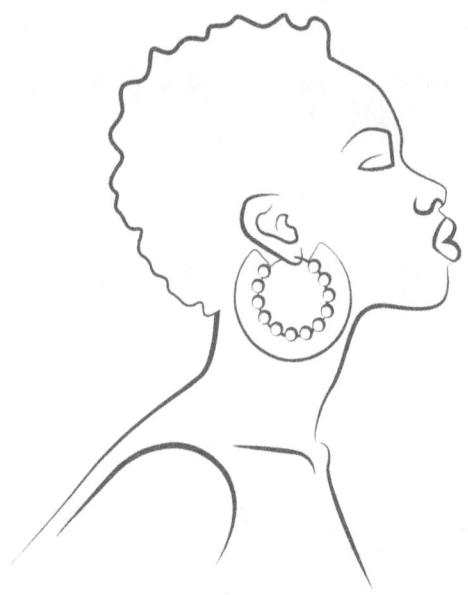

Embracing your natural hair journey allows for endless styling options. Explore different hairstyles like twist-outs, braid-outs, bantu knots, or protective styles such as braids and wigs. Experiment with different looks to discover your favorite go-to styles.

DATE: _____

I will be innovative with my hairstyles and embrace this natural hair journey. I want to try the following styles...

DATE: _____

STEP EIGHT
Embrace Your Bad Hair Days

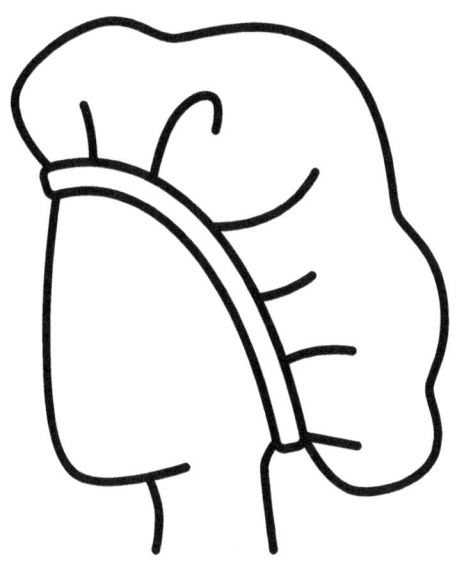

Not every hair day will be perfect, and that's okay. Embrace the imperfections and embrace the freedom of your natural hair. Instead of feeling discouraged, see it as an opportunity to be creative with your styling or simply give your hair a break.

DATE: _____

Normally when I have a bad hair day I...

DATE: _____

STEP NINE
Surround Yourself With Support

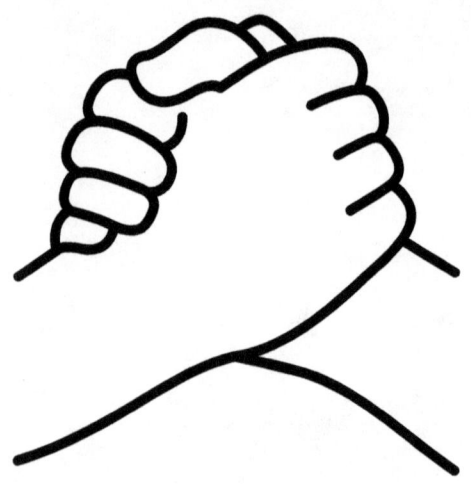

Surround yourself with a community of women who embrace their natural journey. Share experiences, tips, and product recommendations with each other. Having a strong support system can make the journey more rewarding and enjoyable.

DATE: _____

A natural hair community will help me to ...

DATE: _____

STEP TEN
Love Yourself

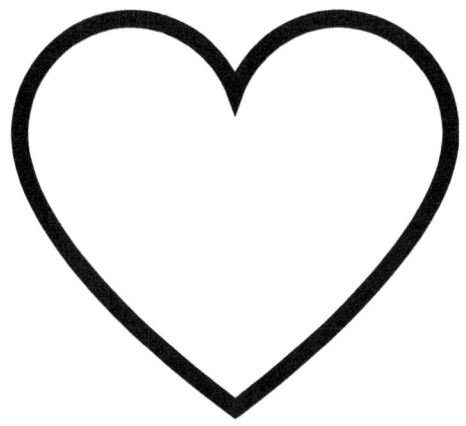

Above all, love yourself and your natural beauty. Embracing your natural hair journey is not just about hair; it is about self-acceptance and confidence. Embrace your uniqueness and radiate the beauty that comes from within.

Remember, your natural hair journey is a personal and evolving experience. Embrace the process, be patient, and celebrate the magic of your natural hair every step of the way.

DATE: _____

I love my natural hair because...

DATE: _____

ABOUT THE AUTHOR

Well on her way to becoming one of Chicago's premiere Salon owners/Stylist Deanna Williams (Ms Dee) is setting the standard for overall healthy hair care. Living by the motto "To Look Good is to Feel Good." She makes sure to go the extra mile to listen, retain, and nurture each individual client. This passion for the beauty industry began at the age of 13, when Dee realized after observing one of her mother's friends as she braided hair, "Hey I can do that"! Ms Dee finally took her destiny into her own hands, after years in corporate America, to attend Truman College Cosmetology program, where she completed advanced training in cosmetology. Once Ms Dee was licensed, she benefited from additional training in the area of Blow-Drying, Coloring, and Smoothing out hair without the assistance of chemicals. After much soul searching and prayer, RelaxShesNatural™ Hair Studio was born, it is the purest example of when your God-given gifts meet destiny. It's one of the most diverse natural hair salons in the world, Dee is always looking for ways to cultivate the beauty industry by attending workshops, seminars, and training from world-renowned stylists. RelaxShesNatural™ is home to some of Chicago's most talented stylists and is also endorsed by ESSENCE MAGAZINE! Her salon is conveniently located five minutes outside of Downtown Chicago, relaxing professional atmosphere, make sure you pay a visit to the salon known for having the "Best Silk Press In The Mid West!"

Follow My Natural Journey

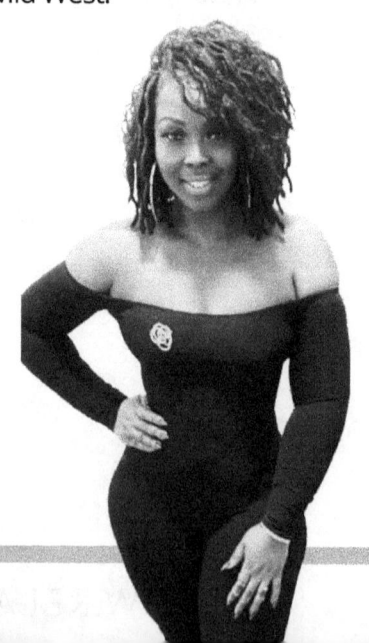

www.ingramcontent.com/pod-product-compliance
Lightning Source LLC
Chambersburg PA
CBHW051949160426
43198CB00013B/2363